MOTIVATION FOR WOMEN

THE INSPIRED LADY

Unlock The Limitless Potential That You Possess

Phoebe Walker

Table of Contents

PART 1 5
Chapter 1: The Difference Between Professionals and Amateurs 6
Chapter 2: *What To Do When You Feel Like Giving Up* 9
Chapter 3: When To Be Unreasonable With Yourself 12
Chapter 4: NOTHING IS IMPOSSIBLE 17
Chapter 5: Keep Moving When Things Get Hard 19
Chapter 6: How To Stop Worrying About Failure 23
Chapter 7: How To Rid Yourself of Distraction 27
Chapter 8: Living in the Moment 30
Chapter 9: Structure Your Day With Tasks You Excel At and Enjoy . 32
Chapter 10: 8 Ways to Create A More Positive Mindset 34
PART 2 39
Chapter 1: **Start Working On Your Dreams Today** 40
Chapter 2: Setting Too High Expectations 44
Chapter 3: How to Learn Faster 47
Chapter 4: The Only Obstacle Is Yourself 50
Chapter 5: *The Goal Is Not The Point* 55
Chapter 6: 8 Tips to Become More Resilient 58
Chapter 7: Live A Long, Important Life 62
Chapter 8: How To Start Working Immediately 65
Chapter 9: You're Good Enough 69
Chapter 10: Dealing With Feelings of Overwhelm 72
PART 3 75
Chapter 1: Feeling Lost In Life 76
Chapter 2: Deal With Your Fears Now 79
Chapter 3: Being Mentally Strong 82
Chapter 4: Creating Successful Habits 85

Chapter 5: Develop A Habit of Studying... 89
Chapter 6: Dealing With Difficult People... 92
Chapter 7: Being Authentic... 97
Chapter 8: Become A High Performer.. 99
Chapter 9: How To Focus and Concentrate On Your Work............. 103
Chapter 10: Believe in Yourself.. 108

PART 1

Chapter 1:
The Difference Between Professionals and Amateurs

It doesn't matter what you are trying to become better at. If you only do the work when you're motivated, then you'll never be consistent enough to become a professional. The ability to show up every day, stick to the schedule, and do the work, especially when you don't feel like it — is so valuable that you need to become better 99% of the time. I've seen this in my own experiences. When I don't miss workouts, I get in the best shape of my life. When I write every week, I become a better writer. When I travel and take my camera out every day, I take better photos. It's simple and powerful. But why is it so difficult?

The Pain of Being A Pro

Approaching your goals — whatever they are — with the attitude of a professional isn't easy. Being a pro is painful. The simple fact of the matter is that most of the time, we are inconsistent. We all have goals that we would like to achieve and dreams that we would like to fulfill, but it doesn't matter what you are trying to become better at. If you only do the work when it's convenient or exciting, then you'll never be consistent enough to achieve remarkable results.

I can guarantee that if you manage to start a habit and keep sticking to it, there will be days when you feel like quitting. When you start a business, there will be days when you don't feel like showing up. When you're at the gym, there will be sets that you don't feel like finishing. When it's time to write, there will be days that you don't feel like typing. But stepping up when it's annoying or painful or draining to do so, that's what makes the difference between a professional and an amateur.

Professionals stick to the schedule. Amateurs let life get in the way. Professionals know what is important to them and work towards it with purpose. Amateurs get pulled off course by the urgencies of life. **You'll Never Regret Starting Important Work.**

Some people might think I'm promoting the benefits of being a workaholic. "Professionals work harder than everyone else, and that's why they're great." That's not it at all.

Being a pro is about having the discipline to commit to what is important to you instead of merely saying something is important to you. It's about starting when you feel like stopping, not because you want to work more, but because your goal is important enough to you that you don't simply work on it when it's convenient. Becoming a pro is about making your priorities a reality.

There have been many sets that I haven't felt like finishing, but I've never regretted doing the workout. There have been many articles I haven't felt like writing, but I've never regretted publishing on schedule. There have been many days I've felt like relaxing, but I've never regretted showing up and working on something important to me.

Becoming a pro doesn't mean you're a workaholic. It means that you're good at making time for what matters to you — especially when you don't feel like it — instead of playing the role of the victim and letting life happen to you.

Chapter 2:

What To Do When You Feel Like Giving Up

I remember going through the phase when I saw nothing but black. When nothing seemed to cheer me up. When even the calmest of breeze shook me off my feet. But I can also tell that I am not in that place now.

I can understand and feel the pain that most people go through. The common pain of not knowing what to do with life when we are at the bottom of that well.

We get stuck at the bottom because we have had our fair share of failures. I know we don't get enough chances to give things the right twist. So we are open to using the chances when we deem necessary.

No matter how hard we try, we always get hit back harder, because we are being tested in the hardest ways out there. We need to do some things on our own because life might not cooperate with us.

You might have heard the phrase, 'Every Action has an Equal and opposite reaction'. I know it I a scientific fact, but it is also a fact about life. Let me explain.

Whenever we try to create a new path, or we try to create a new thing, a thing that never existed before that, nature acts against it and tries to normalize it. This act of nature creates a conflict and it appears to us as if everything is acting against us.

That everything wants us to stop. That everything wants us to fail. That everyone wants you to remain the same. And that is when you feel like giving up.

I know this all sounded silly. But I wanted to make you realize that everything happens for a reason. And I wanted you to realize that finding this story stupid means that at least now you are trying to follow reason and make a logical explanation for everything that happens to you.

But now if you want to find a reason, let me give you one. You are being tested because if you give up now, then you don't have a good enough reason to live for. But if you decide to keep the struggle going, then you have a reason to live for and you are motivated enough to keep the life cycle going.

This reason on its own is a worthy cause to keep going. You can find yourself stuck in the deepest darkest corner of your life but you must always find a way to climb up. Because you had a reason for all your actions when you first started and those reasons have not changed.

The reasons might have faded away because you wanted to follow an easy path. But the path is never easy. It never was and it never will be. It might be shorter sometimes and sometimes it might take your whole life to finish it. But you will always need to keep going along it because this is the purpose of your life that you yourself have set.

Chapter 3: When To Be Unreasonable With Yourself

"When we treat man as he is, we make him worse than he is; when we treat him as if he already were what he potentially could be, we make him what he should be." - Johann Wolfgang von Goethe.

"Oh, come on! Be reasonable." Perhaps you have heard this phrase a million times, either from your parents, colleagues, friends, or ex. The society we live in strongly emphasizes "reasonable" behavior. It tells you not to do anything that makes others feel uncomfortable and which may look as if you're too demanding. In short, don't rock the boat. This may even get to the point where we aren't allowed to ask for anything or simply enjoy our lives. We shrink like unwatered flowers, fading up into the ground with the belief that we are not expected to follow our joy and dreams.

Many people think that it's important to have limitations to everything in life or achieve anything; we have to accept and remain in these limitations. But they are certainly wrong!

If you notice those people who have always achieved what they wanted, the common thing is their ability to break such limitations. They always work towards the things that seem impossible or possibly silly in the world's eyes. They put in efforts that are way too much and unconventional, which is how they break these limitations.

Being unreasonable means doing things that everyone thinks are too much or logical and not accept any limitations. It means trying and achieving something which is not only impossible to do but also impossible to dream. This could be achieved by doing two activities; set unreasonable goals and take unjustified actions. Make your goals unreasonably big so that they always keep you alert and focused. Ensure that you are 100% aware of what you want to achieve and do not waste your time on anything else. "Massive actions must follow massive thoughts." - Grant Cardone. Take unreasonable actions along with your unjustified goals. These actions are what separates the average from the extraordinary. At the end of the day, whatever thoughts you might have, it's your actions that count. Even if we don't reach our high goals, we become much better off than before. The balance that we need to achieve this is a combination of appreciation and achievement. Do your best to become your best and be grateful for whatever you earn along the way.

When It Is Time To Say No To Things

In my previous video I talked about the joys of saying yes to things and taking time out of your work to enjoy life and hanging out with friends. And I encouraged everyone to put themselves in favourable positions where they could say yes to things. However the question that we have to answer for ourselves today is "when should we draw the line and when does yes actually stops yielding benefits and instead could harm our progress towards the goals that we have set for ourselves?

To answer this question, I will bring it back to my own life once again to try and give it some perspective. As all of you know by now, I was working hard in prioritising social activities as I felt that there was a huge imbalance in my work life and my play life. At one point in my life, work was a full on 99% and play was a measly 1%. And simple math would tell you that it wasn't very healthy at all.

But as I started baking in more fun activities into my schedule, the percentage difference grew smaller and smaller. And it became so easy to simply choose fun over work that i actually started spending less time on my work than I did on friends. And similarly, simple math would tell u that too much of a good thing might not actually be that good after all.

As an entrepreneur, I am what I put into my business. And less time spent on my work also meant that I started falling behind on deadlines that I had set for myself at the beginning of the year. I became increasingly complacent and my income started to stagnate. It was at the point that i knew again that I needed to change something. I needed to tweak and prioritise my time more wisely. Carving time out for work whilst also balancing friends and sports for health and fitness purposes.

For those working a 9-5 job, there is a clear definition between work time and play time, but as as someone who is self employed, that line is often blurred. And without proper structure, commitment, and time management, one can easily fall into the trap of simply justifying time off. There is no boss breathing down my neck and that could be a good or bad thing depending on how you look at it.

You see, life is all about constant adjustments and fine tuning until we reach an equilibrium that we can say is the perfect balance. That ratio need not necessarily be 50/50, it could be any ratio that you decide it should be. I decided that I needed to spend 70% of my time on work at 30% of my time on social activities. And my next goal was to restructure my time accordingly. that meant that I needed to learn how to say no or grab a rain check when friends asked me out.

I also had to figure out what kind of work and play schedule would work for me. And the easiest was to look at my calender to carve out blocks of time that I know i would be the most productive and to just work as much as i could. If someone were to ask me out on those blocks of time, i needed to have the discipline to say no and to ask for a reschedule into one of the slots of that I have set aside for play.

You see I know myself better than anyone, and I know that if I scheduled play before work, 99% of the time, I would just end up spending the whole day playing and then regretting after that I had not done any work at all. So knowing yourself and how you function is key here in deciding when to say no or yes to things.

As I became more disciplined in saying no, I saw my productivity at work start to pic. R Rk up again. And I was back on track to reaching my goals again. I also slowly clawed my productivity back up to 70%. And I felt that it was the perfect balance for me.

So the takeaway from today's video is that you need to figure out what your goals are and exactly how much time you should or need to spend on your work to justify to yourselves that you have put in enough work to move the needle forward in your life without sacrificing time with friends. You need to be busy enough to be productive but not too busy that you come across as unavailable all the time. And you need to know who you are as a person and what exactly the balance is that you need to ensure that you are covering all areas of your life and that you are satisfied and happy with that decision.

So I challenge each and everyone of you today to take stock of your time, how you are spending them, what your goals are, so that when an invite comes, you know exactly whether to say no or yes without feelings of regret.

I hope you learned something new today and i wish you all the best in your endeavours. Take care and I'll see you in the next one.

Chapter 4:
NOTHING IS IMPOSSIBLE

Success is a concept as individual as beauty is, in the eye of the beholder, but with each individuals success comes testing circumstances, the price that must be paid in advance.

The grind,

The pain and the losses all champions have endured.

These hardships are no reason to quit but an indicator that you are heading in the right direction, because we must walk through the rain to see the rainbow and we must endure loss to make space for our new desired results.

Often the bigger the desired change , the bigger the pain, and this is why so few do it.

The very fact that are listening to this right now says to me you have something extra about you.

Inside you know there is more for you and that dream you have, you believe it is possible.

If others have done it before, then so can you , because we can do anything we set our minds and hearts to.

But we must take control of our destiny, have clear results in mind and take calculated action towards those results.

The path may be foggy and unknown but as you commit to the result and believe in it the path, it will be revealed soon enough.

We don't need to know the how, to declare we are going to do something, the how will come later.

Clear commitment to the result is key .

Too many people never live their dreams because they don't know how.

The how can be found out always if we can commit and believe fully in the process.

Faith is the magic elixir to success, without it nothing is possible.

What you believe about you is everything

If you believe you cannot swim and your dream is to be an Olympic swimming champion, what are your chances?

Any rational person would say, well learn to swim,

How many of you want to be multi-millionaires?

I guess everyone?

How many out there know how to get to such a status?

Would we just give up and say it is impossible?

Or would it be as logical as simply learning how to swim or ride a bike?

We believe someone could be an Olympic swimming champion with training and practice , but not a multi-millionaire?

Many of us think big goals are simply too unrealistic.

Fear of failure , fear of what people might think , fear of change , all common reasons for aiming low in life.

But when we aim low and succeed the disappointment in that success is a foul tasting medicine.

Start gaining clarity in the reality of our results.

By thinking bigger we all have the ability to hit what seem now like unrealistic heights, but later realise that nothing is impossible.

We should all start from the assumption that we can do anything, it might take years of training but we can do it. Anything we set our minds to, we can do it.

So ask yourself right now those very important questions.

What exactly would I be doing right now that will make me the happiest person in the world? How much money do I want ?

What kind of relationships do I want?

When You have defined those things clearly,

Set the bar high and accept nothing less.

Because life will pay you any price.

But the time is ticking, you can't have it twice.

Chapter 5:
Keep Moving When Things Get Hard

Keep to your goals by putting problems into perspective.
In times of difficulty, most give up.
Don't be like those people.

Difficulties are there to challenge us.
Difficulties are there to help us think outside the box.

Seek to change as you seek success.
Things never really stay the same.
Paths are never that straight.
You always come to a fork in the road.

Think of this new life and realise that thoughts will change how you act.
To have of a better life you must first consider losing this one you have now.

To achieve an extreme desired change you lose everything in the process.
It can be a tough pill to swallow.
It can be hard to see the silver lining.

But if you can keep moving towards what you have in mind,
sooner or later the new life will start to take shape.
First you must be unwavering in your faith.

It will get hard before it gets easy.
You must endure the winter to see the spring and summer.
You must weather the storm to see the sunshine.

The Inspired Lady

Hard times come to all those who seek success.
Your courage will be tested.
Your endurance and persistence will be tested.
No one is exempt from this price.

You will find that nearly all your life's problems come from fear, loss, and pain,
but they are not as powerful as they appear.
They are no match for you if you believe that.
They are illusions.
Illusions because they are only real in our minds if we allow them to fester.

Most of your perceived problems never actually happened.
Most of your fears were phantoms of the mind.
Be prepared to lose it all if you desire a new life.

You must push through the pain to receive the gain.
In times of pain and struggle, you will grow.
In times of uncertainty, your bravery will shine through.
If you persist, you will make it through any problem.
You will become successful.
You must defeat the 3 phantoms to reach the promised land of health, happiness and wealth.

Self-mastery is not a battle with yourself.
Self-mastery is letting your inner-self take control.
The more you listen to your gut feeling the better your choices.

Your inner voice knows far more than your brain can tell you.
Problems arise because you have not taken action.
Force that change upon yourself.

You are like a shark.

The Inspired Lady

You will die if you stop moving forward.
You will die if you accept defeat.

You must move forward like a shark.
No matter what,
Just keep swimming.
No matter what,
Get to your desired location
Get tough with yourself.
The outcome hangs in the balance.

Trust your inner compass to guide you.
Help who you can along the way.
Your thoughts will become reality good or bad.
Remain focus on the good despite the bad.
Lasting success is waiting for you.

YOU WILL MAKE IT as long as YOU DON'T QUIT!
Persistence is key.
Persist in getting what you want.
Persist in fighting for the job you desire.
Never give up even if you get rejected 100 times over.
Persistence always pays off.
You will be given your chance to shine if you keep at it.

Life will throw you curveballs.
As long as you are moving forward, you can still change direction.
Keep the dream in mind as you navigate through this uncharted territory.
No matter what,
Belief in yourself and your vision.

Keep trying to find the best people for your organisation and look after them like family.

One action can change your whole situation.
One action can change your entire life.

You will overcome the obstacles if you keep going and keep believing.
Nothing is more powerful than a made-up mind.

Chapter 6:
How To Stop Worrying About Failure

You and me, right now, right here, at this moment are in the best shape we could ever wish to be in. We are alive!

We think that we had a golden past, where we had everything. We had our parents to look out for us, we had friends to share our secrets with. We had a teacher to gossip about. Now It's just a load of responsibilities that we never wanted.

There is always an innate sense of fear in every human being, that He or she is going to fail at something they never wished to fail at. It's normal. But to give up to that fear is not natural, in fact, it is opposite to the very evolutionary trait of every Human Being.

The biggest myth we Humans have ever encountered is that if you stop doing something, you will never get the chance to fail at it. This is the wrong approach to life altogether. How many things can you avoid with this mindset?

Life is an album of events that will challenge you at every corner. You might fail at every other corner, but you will never fail at every single moment in life.

You have dreams you want to pursue, but you fear failing. The only motivation you need is to imagine the bigger image for when you finally get the chance to rise above all.

You don't need to think about what if you fail or what would people say if you never get what you struggled for. Even if you fail, you can walk away with your head held high because you stood for what you believed was right and what you deserved.

Living means doing the things you love to do. If you had to fall here and there to do what you want to achieve in life, then so be it.

Use your brain. Don't let your brain use you. Act like one unit. Don't let your body dictate your actions. Don't let your emotions derail you. Don't let the fear eat your confidence. It doesn't matter if you fail. You will get another chance to prove yourself. Even if you never succeed at a certain thing, there are countless things to achieve that you haven't thought of yet.

The ultimate failure is death itself. Every day you live is a success. Every second you breathe is a second you deserved. Every step you take towards your goal is a part of that success which will be your fate someday.

The best and the fastest way to deal with the fear of doing anything is to do it anyway.

You don't have to feel good to do things that you desire. It is just an illusion of your brain that tricks you and your body to waste yet another moment that could have been well spent.

Train your brain in a way that when you say I want to do this, Your brain never second guesses you. You start doing the thing in the tenth of a second.

It doesn't matter if you don't feel like doing it. Do it anyway. If you train yourself to act in this fashion, You will have the freedom, most people never have.

No man was ever born who had all the riches and never a glimpse of failure in their life. Every rich to ever exist also had a moment or years of struggle to achieve what they have today, but never did they second guess their instincts. Never did they let their fear get the best of them and then the world saw a new era on their hands.

The best advice I can give to buck up someone is simple but very deep; Follow your path no matter what trajectory it might take, just remember, fear the fear itself and you will rise like a phoenix.

Chapter 7:
How To Rid Yourself of Distraction

Distraction and disaster sound rather similar.
It is a worldwide disorder that you are probably suffering from.
Distraction is robbing you of precious time during the day.
Distraction is robbing you of time that you should be working on your goals.
If you don't rid yourself of distraction, you are in big trouble.

It is a phenomenon that most employees are only productive 3 out of 8 hours at the office.
If you could half your distractions, you could double your productivity.
How far are you willing to go to combat distraction?
How badly do you want to achieve proper time management?

If you know you only have an hour a day to work, would it help keep you focused?

Always focus on your initial reason for doing work in the first place.
After all that reason is still there until you reach your goal.

Create a schedule for your day to keep you from getting distracted.
Distractions are everywhere.
It pops up on your phone.
It pops up from people wanting to chat at work.
It pops up in the form of personal problems.
Whatever it may be, distractions are abound.

The only cure is clear concentration.
To have clear concentration it must be something you are excited about.

The Inspired Lady

To have clear knowledge that this action will lead you to something exciting.

If you find the work boring, It will be difficult for you to concentrate too long.
Sometimes it takes reassessing your life and admitting your work is boring for you to consider a change in direction.

Your goal will have more than one path.
Some paths boring, some paths dangerous, some paths redundant, and some paths magical.
You may not know better until you try.
After all the journey is everything.

If reaching your goal takes decades of work that makes you miserable, is it really worth it?
The changes to your personality may be irreversible.

Always keep the goal in mind whilst searching for an enjoyable path to attain it.
After all if you are easily distracted from your goal, then do you really want it?

Ask yourself the hard questions.
Is this something you really want? Or is this something society wants for you?

Many people who appear successful to society are secretly miserable.
Make sure you are aware of every little detail of your life.
Sit down and really decide what will make you happy at the end of your life.

What work will you be really happy to do?
What are the causes and people you would be happy to serve?
How much money you want?
What kind of relationships you want?
If you can build a clear vision of this life for you, distractions will become irrelevant.
Irrelevant because nothing will be able to distract you from your perfect vision.

Is what you are doing right now moving you towards that life?
If not stop, and start doing the things what will.
It really is that simple.

Anyone who is distracted for too long from the task in hand has no business doing that task. They should instead be doing something that makes them happy.

We can't be happy all the time otherwise we wouldn't be able to recognize it.
But distraction is a clear indicator you may not be on the right path for you.
Clearly define your path and distraction will be powerless.

Chapter 8:
Living in the Moment

Today we're going to talk about a topic that will help those of you struggling with fears and anxieties about your past and even about your future. And I hope that at the end of this video, you may be able to live a life that is truly more present and full.

So what is living in the moment all about and why should we even bother?

You see, for many of us, since we're young, we've been told to plan for our future. And we always feel like we're never enough until we achieve the next best grade in class, get into a great university, get a high paying career, and then retire comfortably. We always look at our life as an endless competition, and that we believe that there will always be more time to have fun and enjoy life later when we have worked our asses off and clawed our way to success. Measures that are either set by our parents, society, or our peers. And this constant desire to look ahead, while is a good motivator if done in moderation and not obsessively, can lead us to always being unhappy in our current present moment.

Because we are always chasing something bigger, the goal post keeps moving farther and farther away every time we reach one. And the reality is that we will never ever be happy with ourselves at any point if that becomes our motto. We try to look so far ahead all the time that we miss the beautiful sights along the way. We miss the whole point of our goals which is not to want the end goal so eagerly, but to actually enjoy the process, enjoy the journey, and enjoy each step along the way. The struggles, the sadness, the accomplishments, the joy. When we stop checking out the flowers around us, and when we stop looking around the beautiful sights, the destination becomes less amazing.

Reminding ourselves to live in the present helps us keep things in perspective that yes, even though our ultimate dream is to be this and that career wise, or whatever it may be, that we must not forget that life is precious and that each day is a blessing and that we should cherish each living day as if it were your last.

Forget the idea that you might have 30 years to work before you can tell ur self that you can finally relax and retire. Because you never know if you will even have tomorrow. If you are always reminded that life is fragile and that your life isn't always guaranteed, that you become more aware that you need to live in the moment in order to live your best life. Rid yourself of any worries, anxieties, and fears you have about the future because the time will come when it comes. Things will happen for you eventually so long as you do what you need to do each and every day without obsessing over it.

Sometimes our past failures and shortcomings in the workplace can have an adverse effect on how we view the present as well. And this cycle perpetuates itself over and over again and we lose sight of what's really important to us. Our family, our friends, our pets, and we neglect them or neglect to spend enough time with them thinking we have so much time left. But we fail to remember again that life does not always work the way we want it to. And we need to be careful not to fall into that trap that we have complete and total control over our life and how our plans would work out.

In the next video we will talk about how to live in the moment if you have anxieties and fears about things unrelated to work. Whether it be a family issue or a health issue. I want to address that in a separate topic.

I hope you learned something in this short video and I'll see you in the next one. Thank you

Chapter 9: Structure Your Day With Tasks You Excel At and Enjoy

Today's video will probably appeal to people who have a say in the way they can structure their day. People who are working on their own businesses, or are freelancers. But it could also apply to those with full time jobs if your jobs allow flexibility.

For those who have been doing their own thing for a while, we know that it is not easy to put together a day that is truly enjoyable. We forget about doing the things we like and excel at, and start getting lost in a sea of work that we have to drag ourselves through doing.

If we don't have a choice, then I guess we can't really do anything about it. But if we do, we need to start identifying the tasks that require the most attention but the least effort on our part to do. Tasks that seem just about second-nature to us. Tasks that we would do even if nobody wanted to pay us. Tasks that allow our creativity to grow and expand, tasks that challenge us but not drain us, tasks that enriches us, or tasks that we simply enjoy doing.

The founding father of modern Singapore, one of the wealthiest countries in the world, Mr Lee Kuan Yew once said, find what works and just keep doing it over and over again. I would apply that to this situation as well. We have to find what works for us and just double down on it. The other stuff that we aren't good at, either hire someone else to do it, or find a way to do less of it or learn how to be good at it fast. Make it a challenge for ourselves. Who knows maybe you might find them enjoyable once you get a hang of it as well.

But for those things that already come naturally to us, do more of it. Pack a lot of time into at the start of the day. Dedicated a few hours of your day to those meaningful tasks that you excel at. You will find that once you get the creative juices and the momentum going, you will be able to conquer the other less pleasing tasks more easily knowing that you've already accomplished your goals for the day.

Start right now. Identify what those tasks that you absolutely love to do right now, work-wise, or whatever it may be, and just double down on it. Watch your day transform.

Chapter 10:
8 Ways to Create A More Positive Mindset

Are you a glass-half-empty or half-full sort of person? Studies have demonstrated that both can impact your physical and mental health and that being a positive thinker is the better of the two.

A recent study followed 70,000 women from 2004 to 2012 and found that optimistic women had a significantly lower risk of dying from several major causes of death. Positive thinking isn't magic, and it will not suddenly make all your problems disappear; rather, what it will do is make those problems seem more manageable and help you approach these hardships productively and positively. We are going to list some things that will help you develop a positive mindset.

1. **Focus On The Good Things**

Challenging situations and obstacles are a part of life, but when you face such situations, you can focus on good things, whether they are small or big. When you try to look for it, you will find the silver lining, even if it is not immediately obvious. For example, if someone cancels plans, focus on how it frees up time for you to catch up on a TV show or other activity you enjoy

2. Practice Gratitude

Practicing gratitude has been shown to reduce stress, improve self-esteem, and foster resilience even in very difficult times. Think of people, moments, or things that bring you some kind of comfort or happiness, and try to express your gratitude at least once a day. This can be thanking a co-worker for helping with a project, a loved one for washing the dishes, or your dog for the unconditional love they give you.

3. Keep A Gratitude Journal

Studies have found that writing down the things you're grateful for can improve your optimism and sense of well-being. You can do this by writing in a gratitude journal every day or jotting down a list of things you're grateful for on days you're having a hard time.

4. Open Yourself Up To Humor

Studies have found that laughter lowers stress, anxiety, and depression. It also improves coping skills, mood, and self-esteem.

Be open to humor in all situations, especially the difficult ones, and permit yourself to laugh. It instantly lightens the mood and makes things seem a little less difficult. Even if you're not feeling it, pretending or forcing yourself to laugh can improve your mood and lower stress.

5. Spend Time With Positive People

Negativity and positivity are contagious. Consider the people with whom you're spending time. Have you noticed how someone in a bad mood can bring down almost everyone in a room? A positive person has the opposite effect on others.

Being around positive people has been shown to improve self-esteem and increase your chances of reaching goals. Surround yourself with people who will lift you and help you see the bright side.

6. Practice Positive Self-Talk

We tend to be the hardest on ourselves and be our own worst critics. Over time, this can cause you to form a negative opinion of yourself that can be hard to shake. To stop this, you'll need to be mindful of the voice in your head and respond with positive messages, also known as positive self-talk.

Research shows that even a small shift in the way you talk to yourself can influence your ability to regulate your feelings, thoughts, and behavior under stress.

Here's an example of positive self-talk: Instead of thinking, "I really messed that up," try "I'll try it again a different way."

7. Identify your areas of negativity.

Take a good look at the different areas of your life and identify the ones in which you tend to be the most negative. Not sure? Ask a trusted friend or colleague. Chances are, they'll be able to offer some insight. A co-worker might notice that you tend to be negative at work. Your spouse may notice that you get especially negative while driving—tackle one area at a time.

I have found that writing down the things you're grateful for can improve your optimism and sense of well-being. You can do this by writing in a gratitude journal every day or jotting down a list of things you're grateful for on days you're having a hard time.

8. Start every day on a positive note.

Create a ritual in which you start off each day with something uplifting and positive. Here are a few ideas:

- Tell yourself that it's going to be a great day or any other positive affirmation.
- Listen to a happy and positive song or playlist.
- Share some positivity by giving a compliment or doing something nice for someone.

PART 2

Chapter 1:
Start Working On Your Dreams Today

When did you get up today? What was your day like? What did you achieve today? Did any of that matter?

Maybe it didn't because you don't have any dreams to work towards, or maybe that you've forgotten what they are altogether.

To have a dream is to have a direction in life. To have a dream means you have something bigger than yourself that you want to achieve.

Everyone gets at least one chance in their life to actually go and pursue that dream, but few recognize that until it is too late. It is too late to regret when you are on your deathbed wondering what could have been. That is when it is too late to work on your dreams. When you have no more time left.

The Moment to start working On your dreams is right here right now.

We repeat our failures every day but never learn. We get depressed every day but never communicate. We get bullied every day, but never fight back. Why?

Is it because we can't do it? No, Definitely Not! We can do it whenever we want. We can do it today. We can do it the next minute. We just lack Ambition!

Every day someone achieves something big. Some more than often, others maybe not their whole life. But the outcome is **not** determined by **fate**, but with **Effort**.

All the billionaires you see today started out with a few dollars just like you and me. They just had the guts to pursue their dream no matter what the cost is. They all had a vision of something bigger. They went full throttle even when everyone around them expected them to fail. Even when they met with struggles that hit them harder than the last, they were still focused on the dream. Never did they once lesson the effort.

No two persons are born the same. Not the same face, color, intelligence, or fate. But what's common for every human being is the built-in trait to strive for a goal once they are determined enough. Doesn't matter if it's food for the next meal or success for the times to come.

The struggle is real, it always was, it always will be. The world wouldn't be what it is today if it weren't for the struggle man has gone through over the centuries. The struggle is the most real definition of life in this world. But that doesn't mean it's a bad one.

Our parents struggled to make us a better person. They put in their best effort to watch us succeed in our dreams. Their parents did the same for them and their parents before them.

This is what makes life a cycle of inherited struggle and hardships. Nobody asks to struggle through a hard life, but we can all turn the hard life into a meaningful one. The life that we all should expect to eventually achieve only if we keep the cycle running and if we keep putting in the effort.

How then do we actually work towards our dreams? By focusing on the things that matter each and every day, again and again, until that mountain has been conquered. Don't forget to enjoy the journey, because it could well be the best part of the trip up top.

You never know what the next moment has in it for you. You can never predict the future, but you can always hope for a better one. You only get the right to hope if you did what was meant to be done today. It's your lawful right to reap the fruit if you took care of sowing the seeds faithfully and diligently all through the year.

The motivation behind this continuous grind of time in search of that Dream lies in your past. You cannot achieve those dreams until you start treasuring the lessons of your past and become a person who is always willing to go beyond.

You can't simply depend on hope to get something done. You have to reach the point where start obsessing over that goal, that thing, that DREAM. When you start obsessing, you start working, you start seeing the possibilities and you just keep going. If you don't get up then you WILL miss the moment. The moment that could have made all the difference in the world. If you don't act upon that impulse, you might never get that inspiration ever again. And that will be the moment you will always regret for the rest of your life.

Remember that your whole life is built on millions of tiny decisions. A decision to just act on one of those moments can transform your life completely. These moments often test you too. But only for an inch more before you find eternal glory. So don't wait for someone else to do it for you. Get up, buckle up, and start doing. Because only you Can!

Chapter 2:
Setting Too High Expectations

Today we're going to talk about the topic of setting too high expectations. Expectations about everything from work, to income, to colleagues, friends, partners, children, family. Hopefully by the end of this video I will be able to help you take things down a notch in some areas so that you don't always get disappointed when things don't turn out the way you expect it to.

Let's go one by one in each of these areas and hopefully we can address the points that you are actively engaged in at the moment.

Let's begin with work and career. Many of us have high expectations for how we want our work life to be. How we expect our companies and colleagues to behave and the culture that we are subjected to everyday. More often that not though, companies are in the business of profit-making and cutting costs. And our high expectations may not meet reality and we might end up getting let down. What I would recommend here is that we not set these expectations of our colleagues and bosses, but rather we should focus on how we can best navigate through this obstacle course that is put in front of us. We may want to focus instead on how we can handle ourselves and our workload. If however we find that we just can't shake off this expectations that we want from working in a company, maybe we want to look elsewhere to companies that have a work culture that suits our personality. Maybe one that is more vibrant and encourages freedom of expression.

Another area that we should address is setting high expectations of our partners and children. Remember that we are all human, and that every person is their own person. Your expectations of them may not be their expectations of themselves. When you impose such an ideal on them, it may be hard for them to live up to. Sure you should expect your partner to be there for you and for your children to behave a certain way. But beyond that everyone has their own personalities and their own thoughts and ideas. And what they want may not be in line with what we want for them. Many a times for Asian parents, we expect our kids to get good grades, get into good colleges, and maybe becoming a doctor or lawyer one day. But how many of us actually understand what our kids really want? How many of us actually listen to what our kids expect of themselves? Maybe they really want to be great at music, or a sport, or even finance. Who's to say what's actually right? We should learn to trust others and let go of some of our own expectations of them and let them become whoever they want to be.

The next area I want to talk about is simply setting too high expectations of yourself. Many times we have an ideal of who we want to be - how we want to look, how we want our bodies to look, and how we want our bank statement to look, amongst many others. The danger here is when we set unrealistic expectations as to when we expect these things to happen. Remember most things in life takes time to happen. The sooner you realise that you need more time to get there, the easier it will be on yourself. When we set unrealistic timelines, while it may seem ideal to rush through the process to get results fast, more often than not we are left disappointed when we don't hit them. We then get discouraged and may even feel like a failure or give up the whole process entirely. Wouldn't it be better if we could give ourselves more time for nature to work its magic? Assuming you follow the steps that you have laid out and the action plans you need to take, just stretch this timeline out a little farther to give yourself more breathing room. If you feel you are not progressing as fast as you had hoped, it is okay to seek help and to tweak your plans as they go along. Don't ever let your high expectations discourage you and always have faith and trust in the process even when it seems hard.

One final thing I want to talk about is how we can shift from setting too high expectations to one of setting far-out goals instead. There is a difference. Set goals that serve to motivate you and inspire you to do things rather than ones that are out of fear. When we say we expect something, we immediately set ourselves up for disappoint.

However if we tell ourselves that we really want something, or that we want to achieve something that is of great importance to us, we shift to a goal-oriented mindset. One that is a lot healthier. We no longer fear the deadline creeping up on us. We instead continually work on getting there no matter how long it takes. That we tell ourselves we will get there no matter what, no matter how long. The key is to keep at it consistently and never give up.

Having the desire to work at an Apple store as a retail specialist, I never let myself say that I expect apple to hire me by a certain time otherwise I am never pursuing the job ever again. Rather I tell myself that being an Apple specialist is my dream job and that I will keep applying and trying and constantly trying to improve myself until Apple has no choice but to hire me one day. A deadline no longer bothers me anymore. While I wait for them to take me in, I will continue to pursue other areas of interest that will also move my life forward rather than letting circumstances dictate my actions. I know that I am always in control of my own ship and that I will get whatever I put my mind to eventually if I try hard enough.

So with that I challenge each and every one of you to be nicer to yourselves. Lower your lofty expectations and focus on the journey instead of the deadline. Learn to appreciate the little things around you and not let your ego get in the way.

I hope you learned something today, take care and I'll see you in the next one.

Chapter 3:
How to Learn Faster

Remember the saying, "You are never too old to learn something new"? Believe me, it's not true in any way you understood it.

The most reliable time to learn something new was the time when you were growing up. That was the time when your brain was in its most hyperactive state and could absorb anything you had thrown at it.

You can still learn, but you would have to change your approach to learning.

You won't learn everything, because you don't like everything going on around you. You naturally have an ego to please. So what can you do to boost your learning? Let's simplify the process. When you decide to learn something, take a moment and ask yourself this; "Will this thing make my life better? Will this fulfill my dreams? Will I benefit from it?".

If you can answer all these questions in a positive, you will pounce on the thing and you won't find anyone more motivated than you.

Learning is your brain's capability to process things constructively. If you pick up a career, you won't find it hard to flourish if you are genuinely interested in that particular skill.

Whether it be sports, singing, entrepreneurship, cooking, writing, or anything you want to pursue. Just ask yourself, can you use it to increase your creativity, your passion, your satisfaction. If you can, you will start learning it as if you knew it all along.

Your next step to learning faster would be to improve and excel at what you already have. How can you do that? It's simple yet again!

Ask yourself another question, that; "Why must I do this? Why do I need this?" if you get to answer that, you will find the fastest and effective way to the top yourself without any coaching. Why will this happen on its own? Because now you have found a purpose for your craft and the destination is clear as the bright sun in the sky.

The last but the most important thing to have a head start on your journey of learning is the simplest of them all, but the hardest to opt for. The most important step is to start working towards things.

The flow of learning is from Head to Heart to Hands. You have thought of the things you want to do in your brain. Then you asked your heart if it satisfied you. Now it's time to put your hands to work.

You never learn until you get the chance to experience the world yourself. When you go through a certain event, your brain starts to process the outcomes that could have been, and your heart tells you to give it one more try. Here is the deciding moment. If you listen to your heart right away, you will get on a path of learning that you have never seen before.

What remains now is your will to do what you have decided. And when you get going, you will find the most useful resources immediately. Use your instincts and capitalize your time. Capture every chance with sheer will and belief as if this is your final moment for your dreams to come true.

It doesn't matter if you are not the ace in the pack, it doesn't matter if you are not in your peak physical shape, it doesn't matter if you don't have the money yet. You will someday get all those things only if you had the right skills and the right moment.

For all you know, this moment right now is the most worth it moment. So don't go fishing in other tanks when you have your own aquarium. That aquarium is your body, mind, and soul. All you need is to dive deep with sheer determination and the stars are your limit.

Chapter 4:
The Only Obstacle Is Yourself

Ever wondered why you feel low all the time?

Why it seems like everyone is better than you?

Why everyone excels at something that you wished you were good at too?

I am sure you have wondered about at least one of these at one or another instance in your life.

These questions remain unanswered no matter how hard you try. Until you realize that the only answer that fits the puzzle is that, it is because of you.

All these barriers and limitations are placed upon you not because you are stupid or incapable.

It is merely because you have limiting beliefs about yourself that stop you from achieving your fullest potential.

It is because you are not trying hard enough to make yourself stand apart from everyone else in the world.

If you lag at school, study hard.

If your lag at your job, socialize more.

If you are obese, break a sweat to lose all that fat.

If you lack some technical skill, learn till you beat the very best in that field.

Don't blame others for your failures.

Everyone else starts off with the same resources and expertise as you.

If others can succeed, Why can't you?

Who is stopping you from flying high in victory?

If no one else tells you, let me do the honors; it's you.

You are the biggest cause of everything that is happening in your life right now.

Nothing is good or bad unless you do or don't do something to generate that result.

Make a promise to yourself today that you will achieve something great by the end of this week.

Envision the big picture and start watching yourself get drawn into that picture.

Take baby steps. take a big leap of faith.

Move one foot forward over the other no matter how big or small.

Once you get past the fear of being stuck where you currently are,

life will start opening great doors to your every step forward.

Sometimes we may take a step back.

Sometimes life throws us durians instead of lemons.

As long as you dust yourself off and move again you are never going to lose.

Don't idealize someone if you are not ready to idealize yourself.

To envision yourself charting your own path, in your own unique pair of shoes.

If for whatever reason you don't achieve that something someday, don't beat yourself up for it.

Maybe those shoes weren't the right fit for you.

Try another pair of shoes, and walk down a new path with confidence.

This could be a blessing in disguise for you.

A lesson for you to strive towards something new.

Something better. Something that no one has ever dreamed of or done before.

If along the way some someone comes and tells you to stop, and you stop to hear them say that to you, it wasn't their fault, but yours. Because you were idle enough to be distracted by others to compromise that dream.

Don't lift your head until you have achieved something today. Don't say a word to anyone about your goals.

Spend more and more time to figure out your life. Promise yourself that no one else matters in your life till you have achieved everything and you are left with nothing more to achieve.

I remember the time my father told me to be a better man than him. The time when I fell off my bicycle for the first time. He came to me and said, 'Don't give up now, as you will fall every day, but when you rise you will achieve bigger and better things than you could ever wish'.

My father gave me his hand when I needed it the most and he still does. But when he is gone and there is no one free enough or caring enough left to see me go through all that struggle, then I will be the closest figure to my father to back me up and give me the courage to get up and start again till I succeed in riding the bike of life.

You and I are capable of riding the high tide. Either we ride it all the way to the shore or we drown to never get back up again. It's up to us now what we want to do. It's you who decides what you were and what you can be!

You will regret yourself the most when you finally come to realize that it was 'You' who brought you down. So don't waste yourself and make a vow today, a vow to be the best you can be and the rest will be history.

Chapter 5:
The Goal Is Not The Point

If you ever want to achieve your goals, stop thinking about them. I know this goes against everything anyone has ever said about achieving your goals.

Everyone says that think about one thing and then stick to it. Devote yourself to that one single goal as you are committed to your next breath. Check on your goals over and over again to see if you are still on track or not and you will get there sooner than you think.

What I am proposing is against all the theories that exist behind achieving your goals but wait a minute and listen to me.

The reason behind this opposing theory is that we spend more time concentrating on thinking and panning about our goals. Rather than actually doing something to achieve them.

We think about getting into college. Getting a Bachelor's degree and then getting our Master's degree and so on. So that we can finally decide to appear for an interview that we have dreamed about or to start a business that we are crazy about.

But these are not the requirements for any of them to happen. You can get a degree in whatever discipline you want or not, and can still opt for business. As far as job interviews are concerned, they are not looking for the most educated person for that post. But the most talented and experienced person that suits the role on hand.

So we purposefully spend our life doing things that carry the least importance in actual to that goal.

What we should be doing is to get started with the simplest things and pile upon them as soon as possible. Because life is too short to keep thinking.

Thinking is the easiest way out of our miseries. Staying idol and fantasizing about things coming to reality is the lamest thing to do when you can actually go out and start discovering the opportunities that lie ahead of you.

Your goals are things that are out of your control. You might get them, you might not. But the actions, motivation, and the effort you put behind your goal make the goal a small thing when you actually grab it. Because then you look back and you feel proud of yourself for what you have achieved throughout the journey.

At the end of that journey, you feel happier and content with what you gained within yourself irrespective of the goal. Because you made yourself realize your true potential and your true purpose as an active human being.

Find purpose in the journey for you can't know for sure about what lies ahead. But what you do know is that you can do what you want to do to your own limits. When you come to realize your true potential, the original goal seems to fade away in the background. Because then your effort starts to appear in the foreground.

A goal isn't always meant to be achieved as it might not be good for you in the end or in some other circumstances. But the efforts behind these goals serve as something to look back on and be amazed at.

Chapter 6:
8 Tips to Become More Resilient

Resilience shows how well you can deal with the problems life throws at you and how you bounce back. It also means whether you maintain a positive outlook and cope with stress effectively or lose your cool. Although some people are naturally resilient, research shows that these behaviors can be learned. So, whether you are going through a tough time right now or you want to be prepared for the next step in your life, here are eight techniques you can focus on to become more resilient.

1. **Find a Sense of Purpose**

When you are going through a crisis or a tragedy, you must find a sense of purpose for yourself; this can play an important role in your recovery. This can mean getting involved in your community and participating in activities that are meaningful to you so every day you would have something to look forward to, and your mind wouldn't be focusing on the tragedy solely. You will be able to get through the day.

2. **Believe in Your Abilities**

When you have confidence in yourself that you can cope with the issues in your life, it will play an important role in resilience; once you become confident in your abilities, it will be easier for you to respond and deal with a crisis. Listen to the negative comments in your head, and once you do, you need to practice replacing them with positive comments like I'm good at my job, I can do this, I am a great friend/partner/parent.

3. Develop a Strong Social Network

It is very important to be surrounded by people you can talk to and confide in. When you have caring and supportive people around you during a crisis, they act as your protectors and make that time easier for you. When you are simply talking about your problems with a friend or a family member, it will, of course, not make your problem go away. Still, it allows you to share your feelings and get supportive feedback, and you might even be able to come up with possible solutions to your problems.

4. Embrace Change

An essential part of resilience is flexibility, and you can achieve that by learning how to be more adaptable. You'll be better equipped to respond to a life crisis when you know this. When a person is resilient, they use such events as opportunities to branch out in new directions. However, it is very likely for some individuals to get crushed by abrupt changes, but when it comes to resilient individuals, they adapt to changes and thrive.

5. Be Optimistic

It is difficult to stay optimistic when you are going through a dark period in your life, but an important part of resilience can maintain a hopeful outlook. What you are dealing with can be extremely difficult, but what will help you is maintaining a positive outlook about a brighter future. Now, positive thinking certainly does not mean that you ignore your problem to focus on the positive outcomes. This simply means understanding that setbacks don't always stay there and that you certainly have the skills and abilities to fight the challenges thrown at you.

6. Nurture Yourself

When you are under stress, it is easy not to take care of your needs. You can lose your appetite, ignore exercise, not get enough sleep. These are all very common reactions when you are stressed or are in a situation of crisis. That is why it is important to invest time in yourself, build yourself, and make time for activities you enjoy.

7. Develop Problem-Solving Skills

Research shows that when people are able to come up with solutions to a problem, it is easier for them to cope with problems compared to those who can not. So, whenever you encounter a new challenge, try making a list of potential ways you will be able to solve that problem. You can experiment with different strategies and eventually focus on developing a logical way to work through those problems. By practicing your problem-solving skills on a regular basis, you will be better prepared to cope when a serious challenge emerges.

8. Establish Goals

Crisis situations can be daunting, and they also seem insurmountable but resilient people can view these situations in a realistic way and set reasonable goals to deal with problems. So, when you are overwhelmed by a situation, take a step back and simply assess what is before you and then brainstorm possible solutions to that problem and then break them down into manageable steps.

Chapter 7:
Live A Long, Important Life

Do you think you are more capable to deal with the failure or the regret of not trying at all?

Are you living the life you want or the life everyone else wants for you?

Would you feel good spending your time on entertainment that might not last for long? Or would you feel good feeling like you are growing and have a better self of you to look at in the mirror?

Similarly, would like to live in the present or would you love to work for a better future?

Do you want money to dictate your life or do you want money to follow you where ever you go?

Would you prefer being tired or being broke?

Do you want to spend the rest of your life in this place where you and your parents were born? Or do you won't go around the world and find new possibilities in even the most remote places?

Would you rather risk it all or play it safe?

We are often presented with all these questions in our lifetime. Most people take these questions as a way to enter into your adulthood. The answers to these questions are meant to show you the actual meaning of life.

So what is Life? Life is not your parents, your work, your friends, your events, and your functions. It's within you and around you.

You should learn to live your life to the fullest. You should love to live your life for as long as you can with a happy body and a healthy mind.

A happy and healthy body and mind are important. Because you can only feel secure on a stable platform. You can only wish to stand on a platform where you know you can stay put for a long time.

There is nothing wrong with working eight or nine hours in your daily life. It's not unhealthy or anything. Working is what gives our life a purpose. Working is what keeps us active, moving, and motivated.

We have one life, and we have to make it matter. But the way we chose to do it is what matters the most. Our choices make us who we are rather than our actions.

The life we live is the epitome of our intentions and morals. We can be defined in a single word or a single phrase if we ever try. We don't need to analyze someone else, we just need to see ourselves in the mirror and we might be able to see right across the image.

The day we are able to do that, might be the day we have actually made a worthy human being of ourselves and have fulfilled our destiny.

If you are able to look at yourself and go through your whole life in the blink of an eye and cherish the memories as if you were right there at that moment. Believe me, you have had a long and important life to make you think of it all over again every day.

Chapter 8:
How To Start Working Immediately

"There is only one way for me to motivate myself to work hard: I don't think about it as hard work. I think about it as part of making myself into who I want to be. Once I've chosen to do something, I try not to think so much about how difficult or frustrating or impossible that might be; I just think about how good it must feel to be that or how proud I might be to have done that. Make hard look easy." - Marie Stein.

Motivation is somewhat elusive. Some days you feel it naturally, other days you don't, no matter how hard you try. You stare at your laptop screen or your essay at the desk, willing yourself to type or write; instead, you find yourself simply going through the motions, not caring about the work that you're producing. You're totally uninspired, and you don't know how to make yourself feel otherwise. You find yourself being dissatisfied, discouraged, frustrated, or disappointed to get your hands on those long-awaited tasks. While hoping for things to change and make our lives better overnight magically, we waste so much of our precious time. Sorry to burst your bubble, but things just don't happen like that. You have to push yourself off that couch, turn off the phone, switch off Netflix and make it happen. There's no need to seek anyone's permission or blessings to start your work.

The world doesn't care about how tired you are. Or, if you're feeling depressed or anxious, stop feeling sorry for yourself while you're at it. It doesn't matter one bit. We all face obstacles and challenges and struggles throughout our days, but how we deal with those obstacles and difficulties defines us and our successes in life. As James Clear once said, "Professionals stick to the schedule, amateurs let life get in the way. Professionals know what is important to them and work towards it with purpose; amateurs get pulled off course by the urgencies of life."

Take a deep breath. Brew in your favorite coffee. Eat something healthy. Take a shower, take a walk, talk to someone who lifts your energy, turn off your socials, and when you're done with all of them, set your mind straight and start working immediately. Think about the knowledge, the skill, the experience that you'll gain from working. Procrastination might feel good but imagine how amazing it will feel when you'll finally get your tasks, your work done. Don't leave anything for tomorrow. Start doing it today. We don't know what tomorrow might bring for us. If we will be able even to wake up and breathe. We don't know it for sure. So, start hustling today. You just need that activation energy to start your chain of events.

Start scheduling your work on your calendar and actually follow it. We may feel like we have plenty of time to get things done. Hence, we tend to ignore our work and take it easy. But to tell you the truth, time flickers by in seconds. Before you know it, you're already a week behind your deadline, and you still haven't started working yet. Keep reminding yourself as to why you need to do this work done. Define your goals and get them into action. Create a clear and compelling vision of your work. You only achieve what you see. Break your work into small, manageable tasks so you stay motivated throughout your work procedure. Get yourself organized. Unclutter your mind. Starve your distractions. Create that perfect environment so you can keep up with your work until you're done. Please choose to be successful and then stick to it.

You may feel like you're fatigued, or your mind will stop producing ideas and creativity after a while. But that's completely fine. Take a break. Set a timer for five minutes. Force yourself to work on the thing for five minutes, and after those five minutes, it won't feel too bad to keep going. Make a habit of doing the small tasks first, so they get out of the way, and you can harness your energy to tackle the more significant projects.

Reward yourself every time you complete your work. This will boost your confidence and will give you the strength to continue with your remaining tasks. Don't let your personal and professional responsibilities overwhelm you. Help yourself stay focused by keeping in mind that you're accountable for your own actions. Brian Roemmele, the Quora user, encourages people to own every moment, "You are in full control of this power. In your hands, you can build the tallest building and, in your hands, you can destroy the tallest buildings."

Start surrounding yourself with people who are an optimist and works hard. The saying goes, you're the average of the five people you hang out with the most. So, make sure you surround yourself with people who push you to succeed.

No matter how uninspired or de-motivating it may seem, you have to take that first step and start working. Whether it's a skill that you're learning, a language that you want to know, a dance step that you wish to perfect, a business idea that you want to implement, an instrument that you want to master, or simply doing the work for anyone else, you should do it immediately. Don't wait for the next minute, the next hour, the next day, or the following week; start doing your stuff. No one else is going to do your work for you, nor it's going to be completed by itself. Only you have the power to get on with it and get it done. Get your weak spots fixed. In the end, celebrate your achievements whether it's small or big. Imagine the relief of not having that task up on your plate anymore. Visualize yourself succeeding. It can help you stay to stay focused and motivated and get your work done. Even the worst tasks won't feel painful, but instead, they'll feel like a part of achieving something big.

Remember, motivation starts within. Find it, keep it and make it work wonders for you.

Chapter 9:
You're Good Enough

People come and say 'I did something stupid today. I am so bad at this. Why is it always me?' You will acknowledge even if no one else says it, we often say it to ourselves.

So what if we did something stupid or somewhat a little awkward. I am sure no one tries to do such things voluntarily. Things happen and sometimes we cause them because we have a tendency to go out of our way sometimes. Or sometimes our ways have a possibility of making things strange.

It doesn't make you look stupid or dumb or ugly or less competent. These are the things you make up of yourself. I am not saying people don't judge. They do. But their judgment should not make you think less of yourself.

No matter how much you slip up, you must not stop and you must not bow down to some critique. You only have to be a little determined and content with yourself that you have got it alright.

You need to realize your true potential because no matter what anyone says, you have what it takes to get to the top.

Need some proof? Ask yourself, have you had a full belly today? Have you had a good night's sleep last night? Have you had the will and energy to get up and appear for your job and duties? Have you had the guts to ask someone out to dinner because you had a crush on them?

If you have a good answer to any of these questions, and you have done it all on your own with your efforts. Congratulations my friend, you are ready to appraise yourself.

You have now come to terms with your abilities and you don't need anyone else's approval or appraisal. You don't depend on anyone either psychologically or emotionally.

So now when the times get tough you can remind yourself that you went through it before. And even if you failed back then, you have the right energy and right state of mind to get on top of it now. You are now well equipped to get ahead of things and be a better person than you were the last time.

You are enough for everything good or not so good happening in and around you.

Your health, your relations, your carrier, your future. Everything can be good and better when you have straightened out your relationship with yourself. When you have found ways to talk to yourself ad make yourself realize your true importance. When you learn to admire yourself.

Once you learn to be your best critic, you can achieve anything. Without ever second-guessing yourself and ever trying to care for what anyone else will think.

If you find yourself in a position where you had your heart broken but you still kept it open, you should have a smile on your face. Because now you might be on your path to becoming a superior human being.

Chapter 10:
Dealing With Feelings of Overwhelm

Today we're going to talk about a topic that deals with feelings of stress and overwhelm, whether it be from your job or from your family and relationships. I hope that by the end of this video that you will be able to have strategies put in place to help you better cope with the feelings and manage your emotions much better. Hopefully you will also be able to eliminate the things in your life that brings your health into question. My job here is to help you as much as I can so let's begin.

First we have to identify the areas in your life that is bringing you unwanted stress and anxiety. I'm sure that if you think a little harder and dig a little deeper, you will be able to list out the things that are causing you to lose sleep over. The thought of that particular thing would trigger an immediate negative response in your body and only you know what they are.

So lets begin by just brainstorming and listing them down one by one. Take as much time as you need for this exercise. Next I want you to go through your list and arrange them according to which brings the most to the least stress. Now that you have this list, we can talk about the strategies that we can engage in to either reduce or eliminate this overwhelm.

Overwhelm can come from areas in our lives that we feel that we feel are out of control. We feel that we do not have a steady hand or the ability to manage this problem that it manifests into something that suddenly feels too big to handle. It could be something that you dread doing that you have procrastinated on, and that the problem just keeps growing bigger and bigger to the point where you don't even want to touch it. It could be from workloads being piled on top of you one after another by your bosses. It could be a project that you undertook that just maybe is too big for you to handle at your current level and expertise. It could be your family who is giving you additional problems that you have to deal with on top of your workload that is just driving you up the wall. Whatever the stresses are that contributes to your problem, know that they are valid, know that they are real and that they are normal.

Everyone goes through periods of their lives when things just all seem to happen at once. Whether it be having a new baby, a new promotion, a new career, starting a new chapter in life, it is usually those big changes in life that we face overwhelm due to the sudden and added workload that we are not used to. Overwhelm can cause us to lose sleep, lose appetite, gain weight, experience chronic stress, and all these negative aspects can surface in our bodies in ways that affect our health and wellness. When we see these triggers, it is time to make some changes.

We can start by slowing things down a little and carving out time for ourselves to be alone and to recharge. I believe great way for us to get in touch with ourselves is through yoga and meditation. While it might seem like fluff at first, I have personally tried it myself and it is in those moments of calm and relaxation that my head is truly clear. When I am actually able to hear my own thoughts and be aware of what is happening around me. During times we feel overwhelm, things can happen so fast that we lose track of who we are. And sometimes all we need to do is to bring back the attention to ourselves. Find a meditative yoga practice on audible or YouTube, or even Apple Music and Spotify if it is available. Let the teacher guide you through the practice. And just let yourself go for that 30mins or 1 hour that you choose to set aside for yourself. You will be amazed at how calm you will feel and how clear your goals will be if you do it on a regular basis.

With this clarify you may be able to make better decisions that hopefully helps you get through your rough periods that much easier. Whenever you find yourself feeling stress and overwhelm, just give yourself another 15mins to be calm and be guided through a short meditation practice.

The next thing we can do to help alleviate feelings of overwhelm is to practice slow and deep breathing. Focusing on the breath as been proven to reduce stress by triggering a physiological response in our body. We trick our brain into slowing down and focusing on one thing and one thing only. This trick can help to calm you in moments of deep anxiety when you feel the world is crashing down on you and you are not sure what to do. Just sit still for a moment and engage in this practice.

Now we have to address the elephant in the room which is what are the areas in your life that are triggering these responses from your body that is causing you to feel overwhelm. And is there any way we can eliminate these stressors from your life. Again as I have said many times before, if this thing you are doing is bringing you such immense dread and overwhelm, maybe it is time you simply walk away from it forever if that is an option. You have to ask yourself if what you are doing can justify putting your mental and physical state in jeopardy. Whether maybe the money is worth risking your health over, or whether this person is worth keeping in your life if he or she brings you much anguish. I always believe that life is too short to be filled with things that overwhelm us. A little stress is good for us but chronic and prolonged periods of exposure to this can in fact cause us to die sooner. As cortisol is constantly being pumped into your bloodstream it can have serious negative consequences for our physical health, not to mention our mental health in the form of depression.

Sometimes we have to tell ourselves it is okay to simply walk away when we have no other option. Something or someone else will turn up that is better for us if we put ourselves first.

So I urge all of you to take a hard look at the list you have created today. Which ones on those list have you been suffering for prolonged periods of time with seemingly no end to it? Could you eliminate it from your life or take a smaller role on it? Always remember that you are what you take on, and that you have the power to decide what you want in your life. I believe you know how to make the right decisions for yourself as well.

PART 3

Chapter 1:
Feeling Lost In Life

Today we're going to talk about the topic of feeling lost in life and not knowing what to do next. I hope that by the end of this video I will be able to inspire you to start looking for ways to move forward and get out of your feeling of being stuck.

Feeling lost in life is a thing that I think many of us will go through at one point in our lives. It usually hits us like a truck when something that we have been working on for an extended period of life comes crashing to an end. Whether that be a long-term relationship, a long-held career, a lost of a family member, or a lost of anything that we have dedicated huge amounts of our time on.

This feeling of being lost usually comes to us in the most unexpected ways when we are not prepared for it. We feel lost because we are not sure what comes after. We are unsure of the unknown, a place we have never thought to think about because we never expect it to happen to us.

There were many times in my life when feeling lost seems to hit me when I least expect it - the most notable one being when started my first business and it came crashing to a halt due to some reasons which I would not go into. That abrupt end to my first business took me by surprise and I suddenly felt lost and unsure of what to do next. Instead of feeling sorry for myself however I took it as a life lesson and decided to find out what my next path was. It took me almost a year to figure that out because I had not planned for this. There was no backup plan or side business that I could pour my time in. For a while I did feel like I was swimming in an ocean with no end in sight. It was only after a long and arduous swim did I finally find some dry land where I could set up camp again.

The Inspired Lady

For those of us who have spent most of our early years working towards a degree that we think might be the end all be all career for us, we may find ourselves completely lost at sea as well when we find that our career no longer brings us joy but dread. Or that we find ourselves completely unsuited for this career and are nearing the end of its tolerance for the job. Or that we may suddenly be fired from our positions without warning. All these factors would be natural warrants for feeling lost because we have set the expectation to only work on this job and this job alone with no backup plan whatsoever. We may realise that we had not planned to pick up any new skills that would make us attractive for hire in another career, or that we may have no idea at all of what to do next.

Feeling lost in life, whatever the reasons may be, can be avoided if we think ahead far enough into the future. When we know the kind of life that we want to lead, the kind of income that we want to earn, we can be better prepared to make decisions today that would not land us in positions where a sudden loss of job will allow us to be thrown into the deep end of the pool. If we start to feel that something is amiss in our career, we may want to start doing some research early to see what other careers we may be able to plan for should we decide to quit our jobs. For most of us, we never want to find ourselves in a place where we have no career, no job, or no income. This sets off a wave of panic and fear in us that can lead us to feeling more lost and confused in life.

I believe the best way to avoid feeling lost is to never think of anything we have as permanent. We should not expect that the same job, career, or even person will be with us forever. We may want to consider starting a side stream of income so that we do not lay all our eggs in one basket. If something were to happen to our day jobs at least we can focus on our side business to tide us over until we can figure out what else to do next.

I have applied the same principle to all aspects of my life to avoid myself feeling lost. I have made it a point to have at least 5 areas that I could potentially work on should one or more than one fail. I never want to be in a position where my day job equals my livelihood. In that way I am forever bounded by 1 career and the fear of leaving or letting go would always be too great, not to mention the uncertainty in even keeping that one job in the first place.

Relationship wise and with dealing with loss and feeling lost without someone, of course I don't recommend you to have back-ups for those. I'm not into teaching polygamy or what not. In that sense it is absolutely and perfectly normal for us to simply go through the grieving process and hopefully move on with life. We may not be able to prepare for this but it could still happen to us. Remember that you should be self-sufficient first and foremost and that sometimes we may only be able to count on ourselves. We can't guarantee that the person we choose to love will be with us forever but we can only hope for that to be true.

So I challenge each and everyone of you to look ahead of you can. Always plan for failure and remember nothing ever stays the same. Do try to be prepared if somethings does not work out and shift your attention quickly to the next project especially with career and finance. As much as you can, don't ruminate on the loss but focus on the big picture. Hopefully with all these strategies I am able to help you not fall into the same trap as I did in feeling lost in life, that you will be better equipped to handle such shocking events.

I hope you learned something today. Take care and as always I'll see you in the next one.

Chapter 2:
Deal With Your Fears Now

Fear is a strange thing.
Most of our fears are phantoms that never actually appear or become real,
Yet it holds such power over us that it stops us from making steps forward in our lives.
It is important to deal with fear as it not only holds you back but also keeps you caged in irrational limitations.

Your life is formed by what you think.
It is important not to dwell or worry about anything negative.
Don't sweat the small stuff, and it's all small stuff (Richard Carlson).
It's a good attitude to have when avoiding fear.

Fear can be used as a motivator for yourself.
If you're in your 30s, you will be in your 80s in 50 years, then it will be too late.
And that doesn't mean you will even have 50 years. Anything could happen.

But let's say you do, that's 50 years to make it and enjoy it.
But to enjoy it while you are still likely to be healthy, you have a maximum of 15 years to make it - minus sleep and living you are down to 3 years.
If however you are in your 40s, you better get a move on quickly.

Does that fear not dwarf any possible fears you may have about taking action now?
Dealing with other fears becomes easy when the ticking clock is staring you in the face.
Most other fears are often irrational.

We are only born with two fears, the fear of falling and the fear of load noises.
The rest have been forced on us by environment or made up in our own minds.

The Inspired Lady

The biggest percentage of fear never actually happens.

To overcome fear we must stare it in the face and walk through it knowing our success is at the other side.
Fear is a dream killer and often stops people from even trying.
Whenever you feel fear and think of quitting, imagine behind you is the ultimate fear of the clock ticking away your life.

If you stop you lose and the clock is a bigger monster than any fear.
If you let anything stop you the clock will catch you.

So stop letting these small phantoms prevent you from living,
They are stealing your seconds, minutes, hours, days and weeks.
If you carry on being scared, they will take your months, years and decades.
Before you know it they have stolen your life.

You are stronger than fear but you must display true strength that fear will be scared.
It will retreat from your path forever if you move in force towards it because fear is fear and by definition is scared.

We as humans are the scariest monsters on planet Earth.
So we should have nothing to fear
Fear tries to stop us from doing our life's work and that is unacceptable.
We must view life's fears as the imposters they are, mere illusions in our mind trying to control us.

We are in control here.
We have the free will to do it anyway despite fear.
Take control and fear will wither and disappear as if it was never here.
The control was always yours you just let fear steer you off your path.

Fear of failure, fear of success, fear of what people will think.

The Inspired Lady

All irrational illusions.
All that matters is what you believe.
If your belief and faith in yourself is strong , fear will be no match for your will.

Les Brown describes fear as false evidence appearing real.
I've never seen a description so accurate.
Whenever fear rears its ugly head, just say to yourself this is false evidence appearing real.

Overcoming fear takes courage and strength in one's self.
We must develop more persistence than the resistance we will face when pursuing our dreams.
If we do not develop a thick skin and unwavering persistence we will be beaten by fear, loss and pain.

Our why must be so important that these imposters become small in comparison.
Because after all the life we want to live does dwarf any fears or set back that might be on the path.
Fear is insignificant.
Fear is just one thing of many we must beat into the ground to prove our worth.
Just another test that we must pass to gain our success.

Because success isn't your right,
You must fight
With all your grit and might
Make it through the night and shine your massive light on the world.
And show everyone you are a star.

Chapter 3:
Being Mentally Strong

Have you ever wondered why your performance in practice versus an actual test is like night and day? Or how you are able to perform so well in a mock situation but just crumble when it comes game time?

It all boils down to our mental strength.

The greatest players in sports all have one thing in common, incredibly strong beliefs in themselves that they can win no matter how difficult the circumstance. Where rivals that have the same playing ability may challenge them, they will always prevail because they know their self-worth and they never once doubt that they will lose even when facing immense external or internal pressure.

Most of us are used to facing pressure from external sources. Whether it be from people around us, online haters, or whoever they may be, that can take a toll on our ability to perform. But the greatest threat is not from those areas... it is from within. The voices in our head telling us that we are not going to win this match, that we are not going to well in this performance, that we should just give up because we are already losing by that much.

It is only when we can crush these voices that we can truly outperform our wildest abilities. Mental strength is something that we can all acquire. We just have to find a way to block out all the negativity and replace them with voices that are encouraging. to believe in ourselves that we can and will overcome any situation that life throws at us.

The next time you notice that doubts start creeping in, you need to snap yourself out of it as quickly as you can, 5 4 3 2 1. Focus on the next point, focus on the next game, focus on the next speech. Don't give yourself the time to think about what went wrong the last time. You are only as good as your present performance, not your past.

I believe that you will achieve wonderful things in life you are able to crush those negative thoughts and enhance your mental strength.

Do The Painful Things First

There are a lot of secret recipes to be happier; one of them is; seek what's painful first. Sure, this may sound a little ironic, but you will be surprised to know that all scientific research is behind this. Behavioral scientists discovered that one of the most effective ways to create an enjoyable experience is to stack the painful parts of the experience early in the process. For example, if you're a doctor, a lawyer, accountant, etc., it's better to break bad news first and then finish with the good news. This will give the clients a more satisfying experience since you start poorly then end on a solid note instead of starting well and ending badly.

There's a couple of crucial reasons why we should do the painful things first. We know that we have limited willpower during the day, and we also know that the most painful activities or tasks are sometimes the most difficult ones. So if we complete the things we find the most difficult first, we'll be exerting less energy on less complicated activities for the rest of the day. Scientific studies show that our prefrontal cortex (creative part of the brain) is the most active the moment we wake up. At the same time, the analytical parts of our brain (the editing and proofreading parts) become more active as the day goes on.

Another reason to do the painful activities firsthand after you wake up is that you would be freed from all the distractions and tend to do these tasks more quickly. If you delay the complex tasks, it will only come back to bite you. Starting with only one task for a day can be enough, as it could lead you to achieve more of them as time goes by. Things like building a new business, losing weight, or learning a new skill require pain and slow work in the beginning to get momentum. But after some persistence, you will likely see your improvements. Behavioral psychology suggests that we're more likely to lead a happier life if we're making improvements over time. Anthony Robbins once said, "If you're not growing, you're dying."

Making slow but gradual improvements is where persistency comes in. It's going to be painful and frustrating initially, and you won't learn a new language in an instant, or your business won't thrive immediately. But when you decide to sacrifice your short-term pleasure for a future pay-off, you will get to enjoy the long-term benefits over a sustained period. Stop avoiding what's hard; embrace it for your long-term happiness.

Chapter 4:

Creating Successful Habits

Successful people have successful habits.

If you're stuck in life, feeling like you're not going anywhere, take a hard look at your habits.

Success is built from our small daily habits accumulated together,

Without these building blocks, you will not get far in life.

Precise time management, attention to detail, these are the traits of all who have made it big.

To change your life, you must literally change your life, the physical actions and the mindset.

Just as with success, the same goes with health.

Do you have the habit of a healthy diet and regular athletic exercises?

Healthy people have healthy habits.

If you are unhappy about your weight and figure, point the finger at your habits once again.

To become healthy, happy and wealthy, we must first become that person in the mind.

Success is all psychological.

Success has nothing to do with circumstances.

Until we have mastered the habits of our thinking we cannot project this success on the world.

We must first decide clearly who we want to be.

We must decide what our values are.

We must decide what we want to achieve.

Then we must discipline ourselves to take control of our destiny.

Once we know who we are and what we want to do,
Behaving as if it were reality becomes easy.

We must start acting the part.
That is the measure of true faith.
We must act as if we have already succeeded.
As the old saying goes: "fake it UNTIL YOU MAKE IT"

Commit yourself with unwavering faith.
Commit yourself with careful and calculated action.
You will learn the rest along the way

Every habit works towards your success or failure,
No matter how big or how small.
The more you change your approach as you fail, the better your odds become.
Your future life will be the result of your actions today.
It will be positive or negative depending on your actions now.

You will attain free-will over your thoughts and actions.
The more you take control, the happier you will be.

Guard your mind from negativity.
Your mind is your sanctuary.
Ignore the scaremongering.
Treat your mind to pure motivation.

We cannot avoid problems.
Problems are a part of life.
Take control of the situation when it arises.
Have a habit of responding with action rather than fear.

The Inspired Lady

Make a habit of noticing everybody and respecting everybody.
Build positive relationships and discover new ideas.
Be strong and courageous, yet gentle and reasonable.
These are the habits of successful leaders.

Be meticulous.
Be precise.
Be focused.

Make your bed in the morning.
Follow the path of drill sergeants in the royal marines and US navy seals.
Simple yet effective,
This one habit will shift your mindset first thing as you greet the new day.

Choose to meditate.
Find a comfortable place to get in touch with your inner-self.
Make it a habit to give yourself clarity of the mind and spirit.
Visualize your goals and make them a reality in your mind.

Choose to work in a state of flow.
Be full immersed in your work rather than be distracted.
To be productive we need to have an incredible habit of staying focused.
It will pay off.
It will pay dividends.
The results will be phenomenal.

Every single thing you choose to make a habit will add up.
No matter how big or how small,
Choose wisely.

Choose the habit of treating others with respect.
Treat the cleaner the same as you would with investors and directors.

Treat the poor the same as you would with the CEO of a multi-national company.
Our habits and attitude towards ourselves and others makes up our character.

Choose a habit of co-operation over competition,
After all the only true competition is with ourselves.
It doesn't matter whether someone is doing better than us as long as we are getting better.
If someone is doing better we should learn from them.
Make it a habit of putting ourselves into someone else's shoes.
We might stand to learn a thing or two.

No habit is too big or too small.
To be happy and successful we must do our best in them all.

Chapter 5:
Develop A Habit of Studying

Life is a series of lessons.
Your education does not end at 16 or 18 or 21,
It has only just begun.
You are a student of life.
You are constantly learning, whether you know it or not.

You have a free will of what you learn and which direction you go.
If you develop a habit of studying areas of personal interest,
your life will head in the direction of your interests.
If you study nothing you will be forced to learn and change through tragedy and negative circumstances.

What you concentrate on you become,
so study and concentrate on something that you want.
If you study a subject for just one hour per day, in a year you would of studied 365 hours, making you a national expert.
If you keep it up for 5 years, that's 1825 hours , making you an international expert, all from one hour per day.

If you commit to two hours you will half that time.
Studying is the yellow brick road to your dream life.
Through concentration and learning you will create that life.

The Inspired Lady

Knowledge opens doors.

Being recognised as an expert increases pay.

Not studying keeps you were you are –

Closed doors and a stagnant income.

If you don't learn anything how can you expect to be valuable?

If you don't grow how can you expect to be paid more?

It only becomes too late to learn when you are dead;

until then the world is an open book will billions of pages.

Often what we deem impossible is in fact possible.

Often even your most lofty dreams you haven't even scratched the surface of what you are capable of.

Taylor your study to your goal –

follow the yellow brick road of your design.

Follow the road you have built and walk toward your goals.

If you want to be successful, study success and successful people,

then learn everything you can about your chosen field.

Plan your day with a set time for your study.

I don't care how busy you claim to be,

everybody can spare 1 hour out of 24 to work on themselves.

If not , I hope you're happy where you are,

because that is about as far as you will get without learning more.

Studying is crucial to success whether it's formal

or learning from books and online material at home.
The knowledge you learn will progress you towards your dream life.
If that is not worth an hour or two per day,
then maybe you don't want it enough and that's ok.
Maybe you want something different to what you thought,
or maybe you're happy where you are.

If not, it's on you to do this –
for yourself,
for your family,
and for your partner in life.
It's up to you to create the world you want –
A world that only you know if you deserve.

You must learn the knowledge and build the dream
because the world needs your creation.
Be a keen student of life and apply its lesson
to build your future on a solid and safe foundation.

Chapter 6:
Dealing With Difficult People

It is inevitable that people will rub us the wrong way as we go about our days. Dealing with such people requires a lot of patience and self-control, especially if they are persistent in their actions towards you over a lengthy period of time.

Difficult people are outside the realm of our control and hence we need to implement strategies to deal with negative emotions should they arise. If you encounter such people frequently, here are 7 ways that you can take back control of the situation.

1. Write Your Feelings Down Immediately

A lot of times we bottle up feelings when someone is rude or unpleasant to us. We may have an urge to respond but in the moment we choose not to. In those circumstances, the next best thing we can do is to write down our feelings either in our journals or in our smartphones as notes.

Writing our feelings down is a therapeutic way to cleanse our thoughts and negative energy. In writing we can say the things we wished we had said, and find out the reasons that made us feel uneasy in the first place. In writing we are also able to clearly identify the trigger points and could work backwards in managing our expectations and feelings around the person. If it is a rude customer, or a rude stranger, we may not be able to respond for fear or retaliation or for fear of losing our jobs. It is best those situations not to erupt in anger, but take the time to work through those emotions in writing.

2. Tell The Person Directly What You Dislike About Their Attitude

If customer service and retail isn't your profession, or if it is not your boss, you may have the power to voice your opinion directly to the person who wronged you. If confrontation is something that you are comfortable with, don't hesitate to express to them why you are dissatisfied with their treatment or attitude towards you. You may also prefer to clear your head before coming back to confront the person and not let emotions escalate. A fight is the last thing we want out of this communication.

3. Give An Honest Feedback Where Possible On Their Website

If physical confrontation is not your cup of tea, consider writing in a feedback online to express your dissatisfaction. We are usually able to write the most clear and precise account of the situation when we have time to process what went wrong. Instead of handling this confrontation ourselves, the Human Resources team would most likely deal with this person directly, saving you the trouble in the process. Make sure to give an accurate account of the situation and not exaggerate the contents to make the person look extremely in the wrong, although it can be tough to contain our emotions when we are so riled up.

4. Use this Energy To Fuel Your Fire

Sometimes, taking all these energy and intense emotions we feel may fuel our fire to work harder or to prove to others that we are not deserving of their hatred. Be careful though not to take things too far. Remember that ultimately you have the power to choose whether to let this person affect you. If you choose to accept these emotions, use them wisely.

5. Channel This Intense Emotion Into A Craft That Allows You To Release Unwanted Feelings

For those who have musical talents, we may use this negative experience to write a song about it while we are at the heights of our emotions. In those moments the feelings are usually intense, and we all know that emotions can sometimes produce the best works of art. If playing an instrument, writing an article, producing a movie clip, or crushing a sport is something that comes natural to us, we may channel and convert these emotions into masterpieces. Think Adele, Taylor Swift, and all the great songwriters of our generation as an example.

6. Learn To Grow Your Patience

Sometimes not saying anything at all could be the best course of action. Depending on the type of person you are, and the level of zen you have in you, you may not be so easily phased by negativity if you have very high control of your emotions. Through regular meditation and deep breathing, we can let go of these bad vibes that people send our way and just watch it vanish into a cloud of smoke. Regular yoga and meditation practices are good ways to train and grow your patience.

7. Stand Up For Yourself

At the end of the day, you have to choose when and if you want to stand up for yourself if someone has truly wronged you. We can only be so patient and kind to someone before we snap. Never be afraid to speak your truth and defend yourself if you feel that you have been wrongfully judged. Difficult people make our lives unpleasant but it doesn't mean we should allow them to walk all over us without consequences. You have every right to fight for your rights, even if it means giving up something important in the process to defend it.

Confidence: The Art of Humble-Pride

There is a very fine line between confidence and overconfidence, being bold and being belligerent, having authority and having arrogance. It is a line that trips even the most nimble footed, but usually because they have dedicated no clear thoughts on how to manage it. Instead, they follow their gut on how far they can push or how much they should hold back. This is the paradox; you need to be confident. You need self-belief, you need to be assured of your ability and sometimes even certain of what the outcome will be. All of those things are empowering. In the words of Tony Robbins, you have to awaken the giant within. But had Goliath stooped to consider David's sling he would have worn a different helmet. The problem was that Goliath had a belief that he was fully capable of everything just as he was. I like to call it confidence without context, or universal, unanimous support of the self. That is the dangerous kind of confidence that spills over into arrogance. Chess grandmasters will tell you that the moment you assume you will win is the moment you lose. Because that is precisely when you start to make mistakes. You become too focussed on what your next move is that you don't even see theirs. You become so absorbed in your strategy that you fail to account for their plan and the bigger picture. It was confidence without context that made Goliath run straight towards to the flying stone.

Confidence without context is an assumption. And the problem with assumptions is that they go one step beyond the rationality of an expectation. Assumption goes into the fight drunk, having already celebrated the victory. But that leads to its inevitable demise. Expectation remains present, it acknowledges the reality of the situation. Assumption arrives intoxicated, expectation arrives in control. That is the difference. Pride is the greatest antidote to reason, which makes humility its greatest ally. If you want to stay in the fight you need to have both confidence and humility. If you want to stay competitive, if you want to get a promotion, if you want to level up. Whatever it is that you want, I can guarantee that the path to get there is a hopscotch of humility and confidence. Every bold step forward must be followed by a humble one. Note that humility does not take you backwards, it keeps you balanced. You can hop along in arrogance, but you will never last as long or be as strong as the one who keeps an even stride. If you strive for something, then you need to start striding towards it. And the rhythm of your march should beat to the sounds of a two-tone drum. Because confidence without context is like hopping up stairs – you might reach the second floor, but you will never manage the pyramid.

Chapter 7:
Being Authentic

Today we're going to talk about the topic of authenticity. This topic is important because for many of us, we are told to put on a poker face and to act in ways that are politically correct. We are told by our parents, Teachers, and many other figures of authority to try to change who we are to fit society's norms and standards. Over time this constant act of being told to be different can end up forcing us to be someone who we are not entirely.

We start to behave in ways that are not true to ourselves. We start to act and say things that might start to appear rehearsed and fake, and we might not even notice this change until we hear whispers from colleagues or friends of friends that tell us we appear to be a little fake. On some level it isn't our fault as well, or it might be. Whatever the reason is, what we can do however is to make the effort to be more authentic.

So why do we need to be authentic? Well technically there's no one real reason that clearly defines why this is important. It actually depends on what we want to expect from others and in life in general. If we want to develop close bonds and friendships, it requires us to be honest and to be real. Our friends can tell very easily when it seems we are trying to hide something or if we are not being genuine or deceptive in the things we say. If people manage to detect that we are insincerity, they might easily choose to not be our friend or may start to distance themselves from us. If we are okay with that, then i guess being authentic is not a priority in this area.

When we choose to be authentic, we are telling the world that we are not afraid to speak our mind, that we are not afraid to be vocal of our opinions and not put on a mask to try and hide and filter how we present ourselves. Being authentic also helps people trust you more easily. When you are real with others, they tend to be real with you too. And this helps move the partnership along more quickly. Of course if this could also be a quick way to get into conflicts if one doesn't practice abit of caution in the things that they say that might be hurtful.

Being authentic builds your reputation as someone who is relatable. As humans we respond incredibly well to people who come across as genuine, kind, and always ready to help you in times of need. The more you open up to someone, they can connect with you on a much deeper emotional connection.

If you find yourself struggling with building lasting friendships, stop trying to be someone who you are not. You are not Kim Kardashian, Justin Bieber, or someone else. You are you, and you are beautiful. If there are areas of yourself you feel are lacking, work on it. But make sure you never try to hide the real you from others. You will find that life is much easier when you stop putting on a mask and just embracing and being you are meant to be all along.

I challenge each and everyone of you to consider adding authenticity into everything that you do. Let me know the changes that you have experienced as a result of that. I hope you learned something today, thank you so much for being there and I'll see you in the next one.

Chapter 8:

Become A High Performer

We were put on this planet because we were meant to be all we could become. Human beings are the sum of their acts and achievements. But not everyone is capable of doing things to their full potential.

Every man's biggest burden is his or her unfulfilled potential.

So what you need to become a high-performing individual in this modern era of competition is to idolize the best of the best.

You will need to understand the real-life features of a successful individual and what you need to do to become one.

If you want to be more successful in your life you need to become obsessive. Start your day with a goal and try your best to achieve it before you head to bed. You don't necessarily need to be on the right path with the first step, but you will find the best route once you have the undefeated will to find that path.

If you want to be more developed in your life you need to sleep effectively. The most successful people have a mantra of high performing routine. They don't sleep more than five hours a day and work seven days a week. They only take one day a week to sleep more just to rejuvenate their brains and body.

If you want to know if you are a high-performing successful person, look into your body language. If you find ease and leisure in everyday tasks, You are surely not standing up to your potential. If you like to sit for a conversation, start to stand. If you like to walk, start running. Get out of your comfort zone and start thinking and acting differently.

The last thing before you start your search for the right path to excellence is to set a goal every day. Increase your creativity by finding new ways to shorten the time of you becoming the better you and finally getting what you deserve.

You will eventually start seeing your life get on the track of productive learning and execution.

Change your way of treating others, especially those who are below you. If you are not a jolly person when you are broke, you can never be a jolly person when you are rich.

Never underestimate someone who is below you. You never know to whom the inspiration might take you. You have to consider the fact that life is ever-changing. Nothing ever stays the same. People never stay where they are for long.

It is the alternating nature of life that makes you keep fighting and pushing harder for better days. That is why you work hard on your skills to become a hearty human with the arms of steel.

Most people live a quiet life of desperation where they have a lot to give and a lot to say but can never get out of their cocoons.

But you are not every other person. You are the most unique soul god has created to excel at something no one has ever thought or seen before.

Start loving yourself. Stop finding faults in yourself. You are the best version of yourself, you just haven't found the right picture to look into it yet.

You want to be a high performer in every aspect of your life, here is my final advice for you.

If you push your limits in even the smallest tasks of your life, if you stretch your mind and imagination, if you can push the rules to your benefit, you might be the happiest and the most successful man humankind has ever seen.

Keep working for your dreams till the day you die. Life opens its doors to the people who knock on it. The purpose of this life is to knock on every door of opportunity and grasp that opportunity before anyone else steps forward.

You won't fulfill your desires till you make the desired effort, and that comes with a strong will and character. So keep doing what you want to never have a regret.

Chapter 9: How To Focus and Concentrate On Your Work

Today we're going to talk about a topic that I think everyone struggles with, including myself. Being able to sit in front of your computer for hours on end is not something that comes naturally to anyone, well not for me anyway.

Unfortunately, this is a skill that needs to be learned. And it is on some level crucial for our career success. So if this is something that you struggle with, then stick around for the rest of the video to learn how you can increase your level of concentration and to be more productive.

So what is focus and how do we get more of it?

The first thing we need to know is that focus is a state of mind. Without getting into too scientific terms, focus happens when our brains generate certain waves, I'm sure you've heard of alpha, theta, beta, waves. But to get to this state, we must give it some time. And the first step is to simply start sitting on your desk and practicing some deep breathing to get you prepared for that state. Close your eyes, just take some time to focus on your breath and nothing else. Feel your body calming down from a more excitable state, to one of more serenity and peace. Let go of any thoughts that come your way, whatever problems that crosses your mind, just let it flow away. If you need to take some time to do so right now, just pause the video and practice this deep breathing for yourself. For those that require a more holistic practice, you can check out my meditation link here, where you will be guided through a simple 10 min practice to get yourself in the right state of mind.

The next thing we need to know about focus is that it requires us to be free from distraction. When we get interrupted in our workflow by distractions such as buzzing from our phones, social media, by other people, or even our pets, we break the momentum that we have so painstakingly built. According to Newton's Law: The law states that as object at rest will stay at rest, an object in motion will stay in motion unless acted on by a net external force. The same principle applies to our focus, when we break that motion, it will take an equal amount of energy to get us back on track again. So to save our brains from having to work extra hard to keep you concentrated, it is vital that we eliminate all possible sources of distraction that will pull us away from the state of focus. It is best that we set aside at least 1-2 hours of our time where nothing and no one can disturb us. Do not schedule your meals or coffee break in between those times of concentration as the same principle applies to those as well.

The final thing we need to know is that focus is a muscle, and the more that we train it each day, the easier it gets for us to get into that state. I believe that focus, as with anything else, requires a daily routine for us to get into the habit of being able to switch quickly from play to work. As you train yourself to be more focused, by first being more attentive to the various nuances of how to achieve focus, it will come more naturally to us if we keep applying the same practice for 10, 20, 30 days in a row. When we make a conscious effort to keep distractions away, when we find less excuses to wander around our work place, when we make it a point that we will do our very best to stay focused each and every day, it will come as no surprise that your levels of productivity and concentration will definitely increase. Our brain's capacity for staying in that state of mind will increase as well. And hopefully we will be more creative and innovative as a result.

I want to give you one more bonus tip to help you get the ball rolling, if you find you need an extra boost. That is to think of the rewards that being focused can get you. Try your best to visualise the benefits of being productive and getting your work out of the way, the time you will have after to do the things you enjoy, if work isnt one of them. The friends that you can see after the work is done, and how much time you won't have to waste being distracted and spending your whole day in front of your computer only to realise you only put in 2 hours of actual work in. Also think of the monetary rewards maybe of being focused, how much more money you can potentially be earning, or how many clients and business deals can you close if you just became more productive. You can even think of the intrinsic rewards of being focused, how proud would you be of yourself if you had actually done the 5-6 hours of work that you promised you would do.

So for those who are struggling with focus and concentration, I challenge you to take a look at the surroundings of your workplace... What can you do to minimise the distractions, and how can you get and stay in that focused state of mind for longer without letting your concentration drift away.

I believe that you can do anything that you set your mind to. So go out there and achieve focus like never before.

Get in the Water (Stop wasting time)

Stop wasting time.

If you have something to do, then do it. It is literally that simple. Nobody likes something hanging over their head, it is stressful and pressurising and the longer you leave it, the more of a challenge it is going to be. Just get it done.

It's like getting into cold water. You can start by dipping your big toe in, then walking away and reconsidering, before putting all five of them in, maybe if you are feeling frisky you'll put in your whole foot. It is such a waste. You know you are going to get in the water eventually so you might as well dive in. Otherwise, you will spend 80% of your time drawing out an adjustment that could literally take a few seconds. What is the point? Just dive in and get it over with. Does it take a bigger first-off effort, yes. But it saves you so much time and energy afterwards. After the initial shock and a few seconds of feeling like your skin is trying to shrivel up, you are fine.

If we can do it with cold water then we can do it with that email, project or book. You can dive right into all that research you need to do. Yes, it seems overwhelming, and that first leap is going to be full of questions and discomfort. Mid-air you will probably be asking what you got yourself into but the great thing is that you can't stop mid-air. There's no turning around and floating on the air until you reach solid ground again. You are committed now.

The powerful thing is that 90% percent of your problem is inertia. It is that first step. It's sitting down, firing up your laptop and starting to work. It is getting past the idea that you have so much work to do and just focussing on what you can do right now. But when it comes down it you must realise that there is no work around for that. You cannot not do that first step. Even if it is just a passion you know that passion is going to keep burning you up on the inside until you allow it to burst out. There's no getting past the cold water, there is only getting into it. So you might as well jump. If you are trying to write a book, then sit down and just start typing. Even if you are not even typing words, just sit down for 25 minutes and type away at your keyboard. Then, while you are typing you will realise that you are sitting down and pressing the keys anyways so they may as well say something that make sense. I don't care if what you type is cliché because at this point we are not worried about quality. I don't care how good your form is in your butterfly stroke if you are not even in the water. You just need to get started so that you are moving. And once you are moving you can maximise on your momentum.

Chapter 10:
Believe in Yourself

Listen up. I want to tell you a story. This story is about a boy. A boy who became a man, despite all odds. You see, when he was a child, he didn't have a lot going for him. The smallest and weakest in his class, he had to struggle every day just to keep up with his peers. Every minute of every hour was a fight against an opponent bigger and stronger than he was - and every day he was knocked down. Beaten. Defeated. But... despite that... despite everything that was going against him... this small, weak boy had one thing that separated him from hundreds of millions of people in this world. A differentiating factor that made a difference in the matter of what makes a winner in this world of losers. You see this boy believed in himself. No matter the odds, he believed fundamentally that he had the power to overcome anything that got in his way! It didn't matter how many times he was knocked down, he got RIGHT BACK UP!

Now it wasn't easy. It hurt like hell. Every time he failed was another reminder of how far behind he was. A reminder of the nearly insurmountable gap between him and everyone else and lurking behind that reminder was the temptation, the suggestion to just give up. Throw in the towel. Surrender the win. Yet believe me when I tell you that no matter HOW tough things got, no matter HOW much he wanted to give in, a small voice in his heart keep saying... not today... just once more... I know it hurts but I can try again... Just. Once. More.

You see more than anything in this world HE KNEW that deep inside him was a greatness just WAITING to be tapped into! A power that most people would never see, but not him. It didn't matter what the world threw at him, because he'd be damned if he let his potential die alongside him. And all it took? All it required to unlock the chasm of greatness inside was a moment to realise the lies the world tried to tell him. In less than a second he recognised the light inside that would ignite a spark of success to address the ones who didn't believe that he could do it. The ones who told him to give up! Get out! Go home and roam the streets where failure meets those who weren't born to sit at the seat at the top!

Yet what they didn't know is that being born weak didn't matter any longer 'cause in his fight to succeed he became stronger. Rising up to the heights beyond, he WOULD NOT GIVE UP till he forged a bond within his heart that ensured NO MATTER THE ODDS, no matter what anyone said about him, no matter what the world told him, he had something that NO ONE could take away from him. A power so strong it transformed this boy into a man. A loser into a winner. A failure into a success. That, is the power of self-belief...

How Luck Is Created From Success

Success and luck, just two simple words with meaning more profound than the ocean. These words are interrelated. For everyone, success has a different meaning because everyone has a distant dream to fulfill. Some people want a simple life, but some want to live with the luxuries of life. "Dream big" we all have heard this; setting high goals for the future proves that you believe in yourself, that you can do it after it is only you that can make you a success. Some people believe in luck, but luck goes hand in hand with hard work, determination, creativity. To earn the victory, you will always have to work hard, and you can't just leave everything on luck. But how can you make your luck from success? One may ask.

There are a few simple steps to make your luck. When you face a failure, don't just give up yet, don't ever assume that you can't do anything about the situation. It would be best if you decided to take control. It would help if you believed that you could handle the situation and fix the problems; when has giving up ever been suitable for someone's life. When you decide to take control of things, things turn out to be just fine.

As I said before, believing in yourself is a significant part of making your luck. Do something now. Stop postponing things you want to do, gather some willpower, and do it now before it's too late. Another thing you can do to learn to be lucky is to sit back and make a list of various options; if you can't follow up on one of the options, then go for the other one. Think about as many options as you can; just be creative.

When something holds us back, it is tough for us to move forward, or when you are stuck at the same routine and are not doing anything to move forward, luck can do nothing about your laziness. Take out time for yourself and decide about how you will move forward, how you will grow. Consider every single alternative out there. After determining what you want to do in the future, seek the opportunities. Whenever you think you have a chance, take action; now is not the time to sit back and watch; it is the time to run and grab that opportunity because you never know when the next time will come.

Successful people are committed to the fact that they want to be in control of their lives; that is how you make your luck from your success. It's all about believing in yourself.

www.ingramcontent.com/pod-product-compliance
Lightning Source LLC
LaVergne TN
LVHW010358070526
838199LV00065B/5853

BOOK LAUNCH SUCCESS FORMULA

YOUR ULTIMATE GUIDE TO WRITE, PUBLISH, MARKET, AND LAUNCH YOUR NON-FICTION BOOK TO THE BEST SELLERS LIST

Jonathan S. Walker

Copyright © 2017 Jonathan S. Walker
All rights reserved.